Community and Environment

**Also in the Growing, Growing Strong:
A Whole Health Curriculum for Young Children Series**

Body Care

Fitness and Nutrition

Safety

Social and Emotional Well-Being

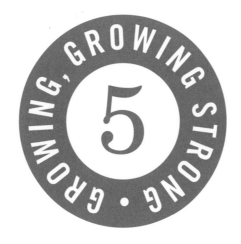

A Whole Health Curriculum for Young Children

Community and Environment

Third Edition

Connie Jo Smith
Charlotte M. Hendricks
Becky S. Bennett

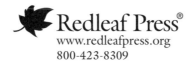

Redleaf Press®
www.redleafpress.org
800-423-8309

Published by Redleaf Press
10 Yorkton Court
St. Paul, MN 55117
www.redleafpress.org

First edition published 1997. Second edition 2006. Third edition 2014.
Cover design by Jim Handrigan
Cover photograph by Alloy Photography/Veer
Interior design by Percolator
Typeset in Stone Informal, Matrix Script, and Trade Gothic
Illustrations by Chris Wold Dyrud
Printed in the United States of America
20 19 18 17 16 15 14 13   1 2 3 4 5 6 7 8

Library of Congress Cataloging-in-Publication Data
Smith, Connie Jo.
   Community and environment / Connie Jo Smith, Charlotte M. Hendricks, Becky S. Bennett.
      pages cm. — (Growing, growing strong : a whole health curriculum for young children)
   Summary: "Children develop a sense of security and self-worth by becoming familiar with themselves, their
home, and the world around them. This curriculum includes activities that help children build connections
with their community and foster positive feelings about health and safety personnel"— Provided by publisher.
   ISBN 978-1-60554-244-7 (pbk.)
   ISBN 978-1-60554-335-2 (e-book)
   1. Health education (Preschool)—Study and teaching. 2. Health education (Elementary)—Study and
teaching. 3. Curriculum planning—United States.   I. Hendricks, Charlotte Mitchell, 1957- II. Bennett, Becky
S., 1954- III. Title.
   LB1140.5.H4S644 2013
   372.3707—dc23
                                                                                      2013025997

Printed on acid-free paper

To the memory of my parents, Nevolyn and George. My mother taught me that a sense of humor is an essential life skill, regardless of age. My dad taught me the importance of love and independence.

—Connie Jo

To Gayle Cunningham for guidance and friendship, and to Don Palmer for always being there for me. And in memory of Nic Frising for showing the humor in life through art.

—Charlotte

To the memory of my parents, Charlie and Jeanette, who gave me life, love, and encouragement to follow my dreams. And to my partner, Connie, who has taught me so much about the early care and education field, love, and family.

—Becky

Contents

Acknowledgments

We would like to express heartfelt appreciation to our talented, hardworking, and ever-positive editor, Kyra Ostendorf. This book is much richer for her ideas, guidance, and smiles—those given in person and those that arrived through electronic communication ;-). Thanks to Elena Fultz and Grace Fowler, interns at Redleaf Press, who assisted in technical editing. We are grateful to David Heath for his initial editing support and encouragement. And, of course, we want to acknowledge all the individuals we have had professional encounters with over the years, as each contact has helped us grow and has enhanced our work.

Introduction

Children develop a sense of security and self-worth by becoming familiar with themselves, their home, and the world around them. They look to adults, including parents, teachers, and other adults in their lives, to take care of them. This curriculum will increase children's awareness of their own communities and ways they can help within their home and environment. Children will also be introduced to sources of help in their community, including safety personnel and health helpers, and they will learn where to get items they need.

It is important for children to realize that health and safety workers can assist them, and that they should ask these workers for help if they need it. For example, in a fire emergency, children may be afraid of the firefighters in their helmets, uniforms, and oxygen tanks. Children may fear police officers if they are regularly exposed to violence or if they live with an adult who is involved in illegal activities. Children who are hurt or who have an injured loved one may not understand that paramedics can help them or that it is okay to go in an ambulance.

Topics in this curriculum include homes and neighborhoods, safety helpers, health helpers, consumerism, citizenship, and environmental education. The activities and resources presented encourage children to seek appropriate assistance (which may prevent injury or death), help children recognize the role of health and safety helpers, and foster positive feelings about community health and safety personnel.

Each chapter covers one topic and starts with an overview that includes suggested interest area materials, learning objectives, vocabulary words to introduce and use (which should include vocabulary words in the languages spoken by the families of children in the class), supports for creating the learning environment, and suggestions for evaluating children's understanding of the topic. The overview is followed by activity ideas. Icons appear with each activity to identify the areas of development and learning integrated into the activity:

1

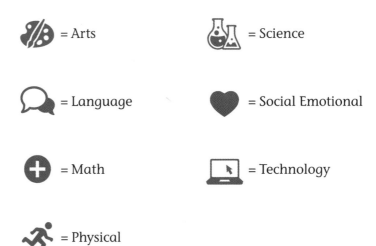

= Arts

= Language

= Math

= Physical

= Science

= Social Emotional

= Technology

Each chapter concludes with a family information page and a take-home family activity page, both of which can be photocopied from the book and distributed to families. These pages can also be downloaded from the Growing, Growing Strong page at www.redleafpress.org for electronic sharing or printing.

INTEREST AREA MATERIALS

Dramatic Play

curtains for windows

a working doorbell

house keys on key rings

sections of water hose for role-playing firefighters

firefighter clothing (jackets, helmets, boots, etc.)

police officer uniforms (badges, hats, blue shirts, etc.)

magnets and flyers with emergency numbers

a variety of phones, including cell phones without batteries

medical scrubs

doctor coats

stethoscopes

bandages

cotton balls

a hair dryer without a cord for use as a bar code scanner

stuffed and toy animals

canvas shopping bags

items with price tags

toy money

used gift cards

Blocks

photographs and illustrations of different kinds of homes

photographs of health and safety workplaces (e.g., dentist or doctor office, hospital, garbage trucks, fire station, police department, etc.)

keys for hauling

place card holders and index cards to make addresses for buildings

safety helper toy vehicles

toy trucks of many types

toy animal figures

toy coins for hauling or building

tongue depressors (or craft sticks) for hauling or building

dollhouse furniture and toy people

aquarium plants for landscaping

boxes for building

Table Toys

a dollhouse

puzzles of houses

puzzles of health and safety workers

puzzles of health and safety vehicles

toy health and safety buildings

keys and shoelaces for stringing

cotton balls with tweezers to move them

miniature dollhouse bricks

small wooden blocks

Art

keys for tracing, rubbings, and making imprints

cotton balls to paint with and for gluing

new unused syringes without needles for squirt paintings

playdough

packing materials

coins for rubbings

price tags

coupons

tongue depressors (or craft sticks)

Language Arts

real estate brochures

paper classified ads of homes for sale

books of house plans

local phone books

chamber of commerce brochures

adult and child eye charts

bar codes

Quick Response (QR) codes

variety of catalogs

price tags

coupons

used gift certificates or gift cards

greeting cards (get well, thank-you, etc.)

Library

Two Homes by Claire Masurel

Jobs People Do: A Day in the Life of a Firefighter by Linda Hayward

Corduroy Goes to the Doctor by Don Freeman

Grandpa's Corner Store by DyAnne DiSalvo-Ryan

Herman the Helper by Robert Kraus

Science/Math

a globe	a light table or light box
maps (world, country, state, city)	X-rays
keys for sorting	recycling bins
nests	real and toy coins to examine and sort
an ant farm	a magnet and screws, nails, nuts, and bolts to sort

Outdoors

a firefighter pole	exercise stations
an emergency escape ladder	a beanbag or corn hole toss
birdhouses within view of classroom windows or the playground	binoculars
obstacle course	magnifying glasses
	toy shopping carts

Technology

a GPS navigation system	greeting cards to record messages
a Google Earth application on a multi-touch mobile device or computer	vacuum cleaners, and clean new vacuum bags and filters
talking dolls and stuffed animals	working flashlights
greeting cards with music or sounds	

Sand, Water, and Construction

toy houseboats for water play	cardboard boxes for creating buildings
small, smooth scrap lumber for construction	straw for building a house
sand castle buckets for molds	sticks for building a house
a water hose attached to a water source	new unused syringes without needles for water play
miniature artificial plants for community landscaping	

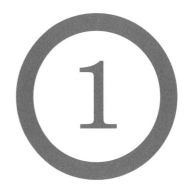

Where I Live!

LEARNING OBJECTIVES

- Children will state their address (for example, town, street).
- Children will identify other people who live near them.
- Children will recognize that people and animals live in various kinds of living spaces and communities.

Learning one's name, address, and telephone number is essential for a child's safety. Unfortunately, many children and families have no permanent residence; for a variety of reasons, many families move frequently. Families may be homeless, live in temporary shelters, or live with different family members for periods of time. Children may have blended families and multiple addresses. Work with families to determine children's addresses and contact information while being sensitive to and respectful of individual family situations.

Assist children in learning the various addresses that are important to them, including the name and address of their school or child care program. Memorizing this information may be difficult for many children because the numbers appear to be meaningless and thus may easily be forgotten. You may need to phrase questions in different ways for individual children. For example, a child may not understand the question "What is your address?" but may know the answer to "Where do you live?" Some children may remember their address more easily if they can sing or chant the information.

Begin with the name of their community, and help them build a sense of identity and belonging. Discussions to identify people who live near them may take place either individually or in small groups. Allow time for questions and discussion so children can share information regarding the variety of living spaces, homes, neighborhoods, and communities they can identify in their area or that they are learning about. In this way children help other children see a wider range of possibilities for community structure.

VOCABULARY

address	globe	neighborhood	subdivision
apartment	habitat	parks	suburbs
city	house	residence	town
community	houseboat	road	townhouse
country	map	shelter	
county	mobile home	state	
duplex	neighbor	street	

CREATING THE ENVIRONMENT

- Post photographs and materials that represent the communities children live in. Allow children to use materials that help identify addresses, such as phone books, mailing envelopes or labels, street address signs, and street maps.

- Invite family members in community-helping roles to come into the classroom and describe their contributions. Ask them to give the children tours of where they work, such as schools, churches, civic buildings and courthouses, parks, banks, and health clinics. Invite family members who have lived in other communities, towns, states, or countries to visit the classroom to talk about similarities and differences in housing, family environments, school environments, and community environments.

- Ask community resources, such as the chamber of commerce and tourist information bureaus, for materials to add to interest areas.

- Go for walks and take photographs or video of the community and special events to infuse the classroom with a community atmosphere.

- Check local policies and consider the specific circumstances of families enrolled before posting addresses or photographs of the living quarters for any child, since doing so may endanger children who are in foster care, involved in legal custody disputes, or have family members with restraining orders. You may need to modify activities to protect children, and you may need to keep materials with addresses out of the view of visitors.

EVALUATION

- Do children talk about people they see in their community or town (for example, neighbor, mail carrier)?

- Can children recite the address or state where they live?

- Can children identify differences and similarities in homes or living quarters?

- Do children talk about pets and other animals and where they live?

- Do children talk about events or changes in their community (for example, a new park or play equipment, a neighborhood or church picnic, or new neighbors)?

CHILDREN'S ACTIVITIES

My Home

Show children photographs of the outside of various types of housing. Include all kinds that the enrolled children are likely to live in, as well as some additional ones. Involve children in a conversation about how the homes are alike and how they are different. Help them examine the details, such as the number of windows and whether the home has an upstairs or a garage. Encourage children to draw a picture of their home, including as many details as they can. Remember that a home may not be a house and that some children may live in a shelter or a car, or have more than one place they call home. Support each child in finding a way to represent their living space. Suggest that they draw what they can see from their home (parks, museums, businesses, neighbors, and so on) on the back of their papers.

MATERIALS

- 8-by-10-inch photographs of houses (single-family, duplex, apartments, townhouses, mobile homes, campsites, recreational vehicles, single-level, multi-level, brick, stone, wood, aluminum siding, houseboats, nursing homes, group homes, shelters, birdhouses, doghouses, and so on) and art supplies

OTHER IDEAS

- After informing families that the children will create a classroom collage with photographs of homes, request that they provide electronic or print photographs of where their child lives. Print electronic photographs, and duplicate prints for classroom use. Return originals to families. Engage children in mounting and creating frames for their photos. Add captions or assist them in writing their own. Provide a space for each child to add their family home photographs.

- Engage children in a conversation about their homes, and have them describe details. If home exterior photographs are available from each child, encourage them to look at the photographs. Provide small blocks for children, and invite them to create buildings similar to their living spaces. Help children write their addresses and put them in front of their structures; then take a photograph of them. Encourage children to add other buildings representing those in their neighborhoods, such as homes of neighbors, restaurants, and stores.

- Play and sing songs related to home, such as "Take Me Home, Country Roads" by John Denver.

- Read books related to homes, such as *Two Homes* by Claire Masurel, *Homes around the World* by Max Moore, *Homes in Many Cultures* (Life around the World) by Heather Adamson, and *A Home for Bird* by Philip C. Stead.

Where Am I?

Read *Me on the Map* by Joan Sweeney or *Where Do I Live?* by Neil Chesanow. Ask children the name of their country, state, county, and city. Show children a globe or large map, and point out the country, state, county, and city. On a map that can remain displayed, highlight or outline the state or province the children live in. Use a sticker to indicate the location of the city or town where the school is located. If children come from other towns or suburbs, use additional stickers to designate approximately where those places are. Show children the states or cities where their relatives live, places they have gone on vacation, and any location for which they tell you the name.

MATERIALS

- *Me on the Map* by Joan Sweeney or *Where Do I Live?* by Neil Chesanow, maps, globes, a highlighter, stickers, names of children's relatives' towns, names of children's vacation sites, and children's addresses

OTHER IDEAS

- Provide each child with an index card–size sheet of heavy paper with their name and address, and explain what it is. Read the addresses to them, and see if they recognize any of the letters or numbers. Sing the addresses with them. Make up a cheer using their addresses, and include hand motions. Encourage children to decorate their cards, leaving the address visible. Make copies of the address cards for use in labeling block buildings, making puzzles, and carrying out other projects of interest to the children.

- Create or acquire a local map on which you can mark where each child and teacher in the class lives.

Assist children in locating their address on the map, cutting out their face from a photograph, and gluing the photograph on their address. Help children see who lives closest to them and who lives the farthest from them. Add to the map other marks of locations that children may recognize (parks, libraries, restaurants).

- Encourage children to write a letter or draw a picture to mail to themselves. Provide envelopes, and assist children in writing their address in the correct space. Give them a stamp to affix. Take children to a mail drop to deposit their letters.

■ Show children a GPS navigation device or Google Maps, and assist them in entering their address to obtain directions from school to their home. Let them see the maps and hear the oral directions. Give examples of how a GPS can be used.

Where Do Other People Live?

Ask children to look through magazines for photographs of the outside of houses to cut out. Talk with children about the various types of houses they find. Once they've cut out photos of houses, encourage them to attach each photo to a cardboard box or some other solid material that will allow the photos to stand upright. Help children use the photos to create a neighborhood. Art supplies can be used to create yards and parks. Add toy people and toy vehicles to complete the scene.

MATERIALS

■ magazines (architectural, travel, home improvement), scissors, cardboard boxes, glue or tape, art supplies (green construction paper, pipe cleaners, aquarium plants, and so on), toy people, and toy vehicles

OTHER IDEAS

■ Provide small pieces of wood, cardboard, sticks, playdough, glue, and other supplies to encourage children to build miniature houses and neighborhoods.

■ Provide many house keys for sorting, tracing, stringing, and trying in locks. Talk about locking doors for safety reasons.

■ Read and discuss the book *Houses and Homes* by Ann Morris. Read and discuss books related to homelessness, such as *Fly Away Home* by Eve Bunting.

■ Go on a walk or field trip to see many different kinds of homes, including some of the children's homes if possible. Talk about the similarities and the differences in objective terms.

Neighborhood Watch

Read *All Through My Town* by Jean Reidy. Discuss things that happen in the neighborhood(s) or city where the children live. Clip articles and photographs from school and local newspapers, record a radio or television story, or choose a video clip from a website that involves area events and topics in which the children might be interested. School ball games, plays siblings are in, new movies being shown, and celebrations may be of interest. Share a variety of information, and always emphasize the street address, the name of the city, and the state where the event took place so that children become familiar with the use of those terms. You may also want to tell the children the name of the facility (park, high school, downtown square, and so on) where the event occurred. When sharing information, refer to any maps or photographs of places that are displayed in the room.

MATERIALS
- newspapers, a radio, a television, a video recorder, and a monitor

OTHER IDEAS

- Invite children and their families to be reporters and share about anything exciting that is happening in their neighborhood. Maybe a new community pool is being built, the bookmobile is making more frequent stops, or new swings are being added to the park. Encourage children and their families to bring photographs of the happening to share.

- Ask a community member to visit the classroom and share with children what being a good neighbor means to him.

- Invite individuals from the media to visit or video chat and tell about the stories they have covered in the children's neighborhood(s). Alternatively, visit the local radio or television station to see what goes on behind the scenes and meet reporters who can give you updates on neighborhood activity.

- Play and listen to the words of "Obsessed by Trucks" by Justin Roberts. Invite children to collect all the trucks in the classroom for a close examination. Ask children to describe the physical characteristics of each truck and to explain the purpose of that truck. Let children identify which kinds of trucks are in their neighborhood or city.

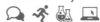

Holes, Caves, and Nests

Show children a toy pig, and explain that he needs a house but is not sure what kind yet. Provide children with straw, sticks, and miniature dollhouse bricks or unit blocks, and ask them to build three houses, one of straw, one of sticks, and one of bricks. When children are finished building, discuss with them the merits of each type of house. Introduce and read or tell the story of *The Three Little Pigs* to the children, and engage them in huffing and puffing and in reciting familiar lines from the story. After reading the story, ask the children if they believe pigs really live in houses made of straw, sticks, and miniature dollhouse bricks. Ask where they think other animals live. Let the children know that animals live in a wide variety of homes, including in holes underground and in trees, in caves, in nests, and in other places too.

MATERIALS

■ a toy pig, straw, sticks, miniature dollhouse bricks or unit blocks, and a *Three Little Pigs* storybook

OTHER IDEAS

■ Read and discuss books about where animals live, such as *Home for a Bunny* by Margaret Wise Brown and *A House Is a House for Me* by Mary Ann Hoberman.

■ Take children on a playground or neighborhood walk to look for places where animals live. Look for dogs, cats, birds, worms, ants, and so on. Talk about and take pictures of any housing you identify.

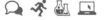

■ Take a field trip to visit a store that sells birdhouses, doghouses, hamster cages, and other pet homes. Measure the door dimensions for each home, and discuss the size of animal that could live there. Take a look at any bedding accessories that would go with the homes.

■ Involve children in building and decorating a birdhouse for hanging at school or to take to their home.

Celebrating Home

Ask children to think about all the things they like about their home and their neighborhood. Help them think about the inside and the outside, the people they share their home with, the things they do in their home and yard, and the neighbors they play with. Encourage children to use art supplies of their choice (crayons, markers, paint, and so on) and photographs of their home to create a book about it. Provide children with paper for the front and back covers and the pages of their book. Then show them a few options for binding the pages, such as with staples or by using tape or binding rings through punched holes. Support children in adding any text for their book. Finally, encourage children to show their finished books to each other.

MATERIALS

- paper, art supplies requested by the children, photographs of children's homes, and binding supplies

OTHER IDEAS

- Read and discuss books celebrating homes, such as *This Is Our House* by Michael Rosen and *Going Home* by Eve Bunting.

- Teach children traditional songs that include the theme of home, such as "This Old Man" and "Home on the Range."

- Listen to songs about home, such as "We Love Our Home" by Francine Lancaster.

- Engage children in creating a celebration song, dance, or poem about homes.
  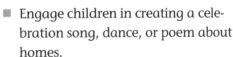

FAMILY INFORMATION

WHERE I LIVE

Young children need to know their name, address, and phone number. Your family may live in a house or an apartment, in a shelter, on a campground, or in some other dwelling. Explain to your child that the word *address* means where your home is located. If your family is living in a temporary shelter, consider teaching your child the name and address of a trusted friend or relative. Your child may find it easier to learn an address and phone number if he or she sings or chants it. Help your child practice saying, singing, or chanting this information in the car, at bedtime, or during meals.

Help your child recognize that your home is part of a larger neighborhood. Walk with your child to a nearby location, and read the street signs, store signs, building names, and addresses on the way. Let your child be the leader on the way home, and encourage her or him to identify from memory the streets, buildings, and stores along the way.

MAKE A MAP

Help children understand how a map is used. You might start by making a map of the inside of your home. Your child can create or follow lines from your entrance to places in your home.

You may want to walk with your children to a significant spot, such as a playground, a school, or a neighbor's house. When you return home, assist your child in drawing a map to guide him or her to the spot and back home using pictures and lines. You may have to make the journey several times before the map is complete.

FAMILY ACTIVITY

Cut out the nine smaller pictures at the bottom of the page. Start a discussion with your child about what is in your community, town, or neighborhood. You might start with a statement such as "In our town there is a library," and then take the book cutout and place it on a building in the picture. Ask your child to finish a similar statement, and add another cutout to the larger picture. Talk about what people do in those buildings/businesses.

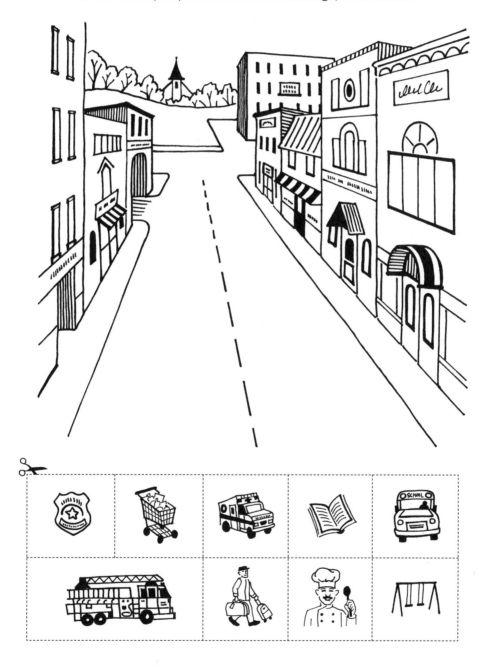

The People Who Keep My Community Safe!

LEARNING OBJECTIVES

- Children will identify safety helpers in their community.
- Children will describe situations in which they might need help.
- Children will practice calling 911 and answering the questions 911 personnel may ask.

Safety helpers are individuals a child can trust to provide assistance in preventing injury or harm or providing care in case of an injury or some other emergency situation. An emergency for a child could be becoming separated from family (for example, being lost in a shopping mall) or needing to flee from a violent situation (for example, domestic violence or abuse, bullies). A child may be capable of seeking help for a fire, a home intruder, a vehicle accident, or the sudden illness or injury of a parent or guardian.

Some emergencies that children and families may encounter will be specific to their situation and geographic location; thus, the focus of this topic should be relevant to your area. If flooding is a frequent event, spend more time helping children prepare for and deal with flooding than other situations. In some communities, children and families are at risk of violent actions (for example, drive-by shootings, gang-related violence). The activities provided in this chapter address more universal emergencies and may need to be supplemented. Without invading family privacy, gather information about critical events the children have witnessed or experienced. Offer individual support, and modify activities as needed.

Who children should turn to for help will be based on resources available in the community. Be aware that some children and families are hesitant about seeking help from law enforcement or other official community resources. Although respecting families' opinions is important, it is essential for children to learn that all types of safety helpers can assist them when they need help.

Help children understand that there are many people who can help them. Teach them to recognize commonly known safety helpers in their community. For example, law enforcement may include police officers, sheriff's deputies, security guards, and military police. Other examples are firefighters, traffic crossing guards, and paramedics. In many communities, children may be familiar with and trust specific individuals, such as their mail carrier and garbage collector. Work with families, and encourage children to identify individuals who can help them if they need it. For example, teach children that if they are lost in a shopping mall, they can ask a store clerk or a mom with children for help.

Individuals, organizations, and businesses related to emergency situations could be included in classroom curriculum. For example, there are businesses that provide supplies for first responders, such as firefighters, paramedics, and law enforcement. After an event such as a fire or flood, volunteers, insurance companies, construction workers, and cleaning businesses provide cleanup and repair services to make the area safe.

In almost every community, calling 911 is the fastest way to get help. Many communities have Enhanced 911; this service immediately identifies the location (address) from which a call is made. This service is not available in all areas, and it does not always provide the location of cell phone calls. Teach children their name and address so they can provide that if needed (see activities in chapter 1). Some families may not have a permanent address, and a child may need to call from somewhere other than home, so also teach children to observe and describe their location. For example, they may be able to describe a nearby building, such as a school or a store. Some children may be able to read street signs or names on buildings.

Be aware that not all children have ready access to telephones and cell phones; nevertheless, they need to practice calling 911 from a variety of different types of phones. Note: When discussing fire, be sure to emphasize getting out of the burning house and then calling 911 from a cell phone or from a neighbor's house.

VOCABULARY

ambulance	detective	game warden	lifeguard
border patrol	dispatcher/ operator	garbage	military police
crossing guard		Homeland Security	National Guard
deputy	firefighter		911

paramedic	Red Cross	search and rescue	sheriff
park ranger	sanitation		siren
police officer	sea rescuer	security guard	

CREATING THE ENVIRONMENT

- Include many kinds of telephones and cell phones on which children can practice. (Remove batteries from cell phones before using them for practice.) Check local emergency facilities to see if a 911 simulation is available for loan to help children become comfortable with using this service.

- Provide photographs and equipment related to the various safety helper roles for children to view and incorporate into their role play.

- Extend learning by inviting guest speakers who have safety roles, watching video clips of safety helpers in action, and taking field trips to visit the safety-related environments of guests and other safety helpers.

EVALUATION

- Do children role-play various safety helpers?

- During conversations, are children talking about safety helpers?

- Do children practice dialing 911 (on an unconnected phone)?

- During role playing, can children answer questions related to a 911 call?

- Do children discuss situations when they have seen safety helpers in action?

CHILDREN'S ACTIVITIES

Solving the Safety Puzzle

In small groups, give each child a piece of a puzzle that represents a safety helper in your community. Tell children to work on the puzzle together, and explain that safety workers have to work together to help people. Ask them what they know about the helper in their puzzle. Help children gather information related to this worker by showing them books and photographs, playing songs, and talking about when people may need the helper. Assist children in preparing and sharing information about that safety helper with the other children. Take photographs of children giving their report to include in a class book about safety helpers, send copies of the photos to the safety helpers represented, and send copies to the local newspaper and television station. Remember to obtain parental permission prior to using their child's image or name for media purposes, including social media such as Facebook.

MATERIALS

- puzzles of safety helpers in your community (firefighter, police officer, paramedic, crossing guard, lifeguard, sea rescuer, park ranger, National Guard member, Red Cross volunteer, sanitation worker, and so on), a camera, and books and music about safety helpers

OTHER IDEAS

- Show children toy safety vehicles and worker figures to represent safety helpers in the community, and ask what they know about each. Clarify as needed to ensure that shared information is correct. Show children a local map, and place each vehicle and figure in the appropriate space to represent their work station. Discuss the distance each is from the others and where they are in relation to the school and their homes.

- Obtain photographs of real people who are safety workers in the community, mount them on cardboard, and involve children in making puzzles, memory games, and bingo cards to use in the table toy interest area.

- Invite any family members who are safety workers to visit and share about their jobs, or invite family members to share stories about when they needed safety helpers and how they were helpful to their family.

■ Use "The Ambulance" by Jane Murphy to play and move like emergency vehicles. Talk with the children about vehicles used by safety helpers. Be sure to include safety vehicles that may be overlooked, such as snow-plows and tow trucks. Play other related songs from the *Cars, Trucks, and Trains* album by Jane Murphy, such as "Lizzie the Snowplow" and "The Strongest Tow Truck in the World."

Safety Community

Show children a solid-color plastic tablecloth. With a permanent marker, draw a main road down the middle and add side roads. Place toy safety vehicles and worker figures on the land beside the roads. Ask children to identify each type of safety helper as you place them. See if children can explain when they may need help from each type of safety helper. Point out that these safety helpers do not have buildings for their vehicles or for them to work at. Show photographs of various safety helper buildings (fire station, police station, hospital, health department, and so on), and encourage children to describe what they see. Involve children in selecting appropriate size boxes and art supplies to create a building for each safety helper and his vehicle. Assist children in placing the building on a lot, labeling each building, and moving the appropriate toy vehicles and people into their building. Leave the safety community available for children to continue to build and play with.

MATERIALS

■ a solid-color plastic tablecloth, a permanent marker, safety helper figures, safety helper vehicles, photographs of safety helper buildings, boxes, and art supplies

OTHER IDEAS

■ Invite people who are emergency and safety workers to visit and explain about their services. Consider workers appropriate for your specific community (park rangers, military police, border patrol, water patrol, game wardens, lifeguards, and on on). Remember that many less well-known safety personnel work to keep our air and water clean and to ensure hazardous waste is properly handled. Ask the guests to show photographs, special clothes, equipment, and tools used on the job.

■ Play and listen to the words of songs about workers who help keep us safe, such as "She's a Yellow Reflector" and "She Sits" by Justin Roberts.

■ Read and discuss books that include a variety of community safety workers and volunteers, such as *Helpers in My Community* by Bobbie Kalman, *Whose Hat Is This? A Look at Hats Workers Wear—Hard, Tall, and Shiny* by Sharon Katz Cooper, *Whose Tools Are These? A Look at Tools Workers Use—Big, Sharp, and Smooth* by Sharon

Katz Cooper, *School Bus Drivers* by Dee Ready, and *Sanitation Workers* by Janet Piehl.

■ Provide the dress-up clothes and props of various safety workers, and invite children to identify and try on the clothes for various situations you introduce and then role-play the situations.

Fighting Fire Field Trip

Show children a photograph of a fire truck, and determine what they know about it. Let them know that they will be going on a field trip to the local fire station. Show photographs or a video clip of what children may see on the field trip, including the fire trucks, uniforms and emergency gear, poles, water hoses, ladders, and rescue equipment. Let them know that they may hear a siren. Help children identify questions they may want to ask. While at the fire station, encourage children to draw, trace, or do a rubbing of interesting things they see. Take a video of the experience for children to review and talk about and for their family members to watch. Contact the local media to see if they can cover the trip. Coverage will help the community learn about your class and call attention to fire prevention. Remember to obtain parent permission prior to their child's image or name being included for media purposes, including social media such as Facebook.

MATERIALS
- a photograph of a fire truck, photographs or a video clip of a fire station and firefighting equipment, paper, pencils, a video camera, and a video monitor

OTHER IDEAS
- As a thank-you to the fire station, assist children in making a class book to show what they learned, and send it to the firefighters. Ask each child what she saw and learned. Use children's names as you write the book. (Allie and Sam learned that firefighters wear great big boots.) Involve children in illustrating the book.

- Encourage children to represent what they saw during the field trip through art, construction, or dramatic play. Provide supporting materials and guidance.

- Read and discuss books related to firefighters, such as *Fire Fighters* by Dee Ready, *Jobs People Do: A Day in the Life of a Firefighter* by Linda Hayward, and *"Fire! Fire!" Said Mrs. McGuire* by Bill Martin Jr.

- Let children know that when a fire alarm call comes in, firefighters must quickly put on their special clothes and equipment. Provide boots (rain or snow) and clothes (snowsuit or jumpsuit and raincoat) to simulate what firefighters wear. Add a backpack, mask, and other supplies to enhance the experience. Let each child ring a bell while dressed up and let another child use a stopwatch and click it when the bell is rung.

Encourage children to practice getting dressed quickly.

Police Please

Before this activity, take photographs of many police officers in the community, representing as much diversity (race, ethnicity, age, physical build, uniforms, and so on) as possible, and create a slide show. Introduce the slide show, and ask children what they think the police officers will look like. Tell children to watch for all the different ways police officers can look. Let children ask questions or share during the show.

MATERIALS
- a camera and a monitor for viewing digital photographs

OTHER IDEAS

- Guide children in creating a thank-you letter and illustrating it for the police officers who agreed to include their picture in the class slide show. Help children use the camera and computer to create a slide show of themselves to send with the thank-you letter.

- Tell children that one of the many things a police officer does is watch closely to be sure everyone is safe, and this is sometimes called surveillance. Provide binoculars, a camera, and a notebook and pencil or a digital recorder for children to conduct a surveillance of activity in the classroom, in the parking lot from a distance, or out the window. Ask for a report at the end of each surveillance. Rotate who is conducting the surveillance so that everyone who wants gets a chance.

- Explain that people who work in police jobs must be strong and able to pass a physical fitness test. Involve children in practicing some of the police officer requirements, such as doing sit-ups and push-ups and running, jumping, and climbing. Set up an obstacle course with exercise stops along the way. Let children time themselves and keep records to check for improvement.

- Read and discuss books related to law enforcement, such as *Police Officers* by Dee Ready, *Police Officers on Patrol* by Kersten Hamilton, and *Park Rangers* by Mary Firestone.

Arrival of the Ambulance

Ask if children have had any experiences with emergency medical technicians (EMTs), paramedics, or ambulances. Let them tell their stories. Show children the calendar, and explain when the paramedics will visit the classroom. Ask the paramedics to share with the children what they do, to show any of the tools they use, and to let the children tour the ambulance. Take photographs of the visit to show children later, and ask what they remember. Share the photos with the children's families. Send some of the photos and a story to the local news media. Remember to obtain parent permission prior to their child's image or name being included for media purposes, including social media such as Facebook. Alternatively, invite a paramedic to video chat with the class and give an ambulance tour and answer questions via a video chat program.

MATERIALS
- a camera and a calendar or video chat capability

OTHER IDEAS

- Read *Madeline* by Ludwig Bemelmans and *Please Don't Dance in My Ambulance* by Barry Bachenheimer.

- Tell children that people who drive an ambulance must remain safe while traveling very fast to get to those in need of help. Encourage children to run fast and to increase their speed through practice. Provide a stopwatch and encourage children to work in pairs to practice and check their speed.

- Encourage children to build an ambulance from a large walk-in cardboard box, and encourage them to add details based on their visit inside an ambulance and their review of photographs. Leave the cardboard ambulance available inside or out for continued role play.

- Show children photographs of stretchers and gurneys, and explain how they are used by people who work in ambulances and hospitals to help move people who cannot move by themselves. Assist children in making a stretcher to use with the classroom dolls.

We've Got Your Number

Draw a large "911" with chalk on a sidewalk or tricycle path. Explain that this is the number a lot of people call on the telephone if they need help from firefighters, police officers, or an ambulance. Tell them they can practice on the play phones in the classroom later. Encourage children to interact with the 911 you have written on the sidewalk in these and other ways: walk on it, jump over it, tiptoe on it, walk backwards on it, push a car on it, roll a ball on it, dance on it, trace over it with more chalk, sing to it, tell it a story, and tell it good-bye and go inside.

MATERIALS

- chalk and pavement or other space on which to write 911 with chalk

OTHER IDEAS

- Let children select any material available (blocks, beads, scarves, lids, artificial flowers, tissue paper, playdough, paint, yarn) and make a 911. Suggest that each child be original and use something different. Take a picture of each 911 creation to make a "911 Book."

- Visit a store that sells telephones, including cellular phones, to see the wide variety. Alternatively, set up a telephone store interest area in the classroom. Help children locate 911 on many different phones. Remove batteries from cell phones prior to practicing emergency calls.

- Invite a 911 operator or dispatcher to talk with children in person or by conference call to explain his job, give examples of when it is appropriate to call 911, and answer their questions.

- Invite someone who has called 911 before to share that experience with the children. Ask the guest to explain why 911 was called and tell which safety helpers assisted.

FAMILY INFORMATION

THE PEOPLE WHO KEEP MY COMMUNITY SAFE!

Safety helpers are individuals whom a child can trust to provide assistance with preventing injury and to provide care in case of injury or some other emergency situation. Help your child identify safety helpers in your community, such as police officers, firefighters, traffic crossing guards, military police, security guards, and paramedics.

In many communities, children may be familiar with and trust specific individuals, such as their mail carrier, garbage collector, janitor, or clerk in a nearby store. These individuals can also be safety helpers.

Tell your child that if you get separated and cannot find one another in a store, he or she should stay in the store because you will be looking for her or him! Instruct your child to ask a store clerk or another parent with children to help find you.

Children need to understand that there are people who can help them. Talk with your child about whom you trust to help them.

911

In most communities, calling 911 is the fastest way to get help. Teach your child to recognize these numbers—both as individual numbers and together—and how to dial them from a variety of telephones and cell phones. Practice using a cell phone with the battery removed, or use toy telephones. Pretend to be the 911 operator, and with your child practice asking and answering questions.

FAMILY ACTIVITY

Assist your child in circling, pointing to, coloring, or cutting out the picture in each row that does not belong with the rest. Discuss the type of jobs depicted by each set and who does that in your community or town.

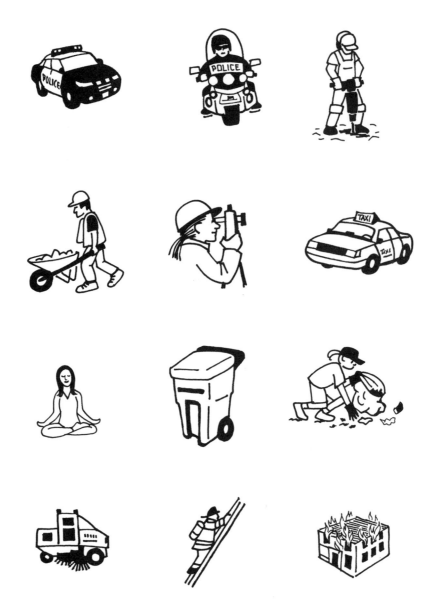

The People Who Help My Body Stay Well!

LEARNING OBJECTIVES

- Children will identify various people who are health helpers.
- Children will recognize places where doctors, nurses, and other health personnel work.
- Children will communicate why people might need to see a doctor or nurse, including for preventive care (for example, immunization).

The American Academy of Pediatrics believes that every child deserves a medical home: a trusting partnership between the parent/guardian, the child, and the pediatric primary health care team. A medical home is a place where the child's primary care provider (for example, pediatrician) knows the child's health history, listens to the concerns of the parent or guardian and the child, treats the child with compassion, has an understanding of the child's strengths, and develops a care plan with the family when needed. The primary care provider also respects and honors the family's culture and traditions, which can vary greatly among families. Primary care providers can help families and their children access and coordinate specialty care, other health care and educational services, in-home and out-of-home care, family support, and other community services that are important to child health and well-being.

Help families understand the importance of having a medical home, and help children develop the confidence and communication skills to talk with their health care provider. When children are familiar with their health care provider (for example, doctor, clinic staff), they will be more likely to tell the provider about any problems (for example, pain) and to ask questions. Children can learn to take an active role in their own health care.

Prevent the spread of disease through the use of established procedures. For example, procedures should clearly state the policy for immunization. All children and adults should have up-to-date immunizations; the only exceptions should be made for documented medical or religious reasons. Review and familiarize staff and families with the written policy and procedures for handling illness, including exclusion for communicable diseases, to better ensure the health of enrolled children, families, and staff.

Work with families to identify and support the individual needs of each child, and build on the health care experiences of each child. When gathering materials or deciding on field trips and guest speakers, include doctors and nurses from many specialties, lab technicians, paramedics, health educators, dentists, eye doctors, and school nurses. Try to include some medical specialties that might be less familiar, such as chiropractors, acupuncturists, and podiatrists. Remember family pets, and invite a veterinarian or other pet care specialist to visit! Information provided by guests should contain references and facts regarding where these people work, such as in a doctor's office, school, hospital, clinic, dental trailer, or health department. Provide opportunities for health care workers to visit the classroom as guest speakers so that children can see them in a familiar environment. Extend invitations to family members in the health care field to be guest speakers. Later provide opportunities for seeing the same professionals, and others, in their various health-related environments by going on field trips or through video chats.

As children explore the roles of health care professionals and hear about the work they do, talk about occasions when this type of help might be needed. Present the topic honestly, but be careful not to frighten the children. Allow ample time for them to process, role-play, and ask questions.

VOCABULARY

acupuncturist	healthy	paramedic
chiropractor	hospital	pediatrician
communicable	illness	physician
dental trailer	immunization	podiatrist
dentist	lab technician	sick
doctor	medical	symptom
health department clinic	nurse	veterinarian
health educator	optometrist	well

CREATING THE ENVIRONMENT

- Expose children to materials and equipment related to health care fields, such as uniforms, stethoscopes, bandages, cotton balls, and eye charts.

- Extend learning by inviting a variety of health-related guest speakers of varying gender, race, and ethnicity; by taking field trips to places where health care is conducted; or by watching video clips of health care professionals on location.

EVALUATION

- During role play, do children act out health-related issues?

- During conversation, do children use health-related vocabulary?

- Do children role-play various health helpers (for example, doctor with stethoscope, lab tech pricking finger)?

- Do children describe places they have seen a doctor, nurse, or other health helper (for example, walk-in clinic, hospital, immunization event in shopping center)?

- Do children role-play or talk about taking or giving immunizations?

CHILDREN'S ACTIVITIES

Roll a Helper

Involve children in gluing a photocopy of a photograph or an illustration of one health helper (doctor, nurse, dentist, dental hygienist, optometrist, or other) on each side of several square boxes. Once the pictures on all boxes have dried, invite children to roll their cubes to see which worker shows up on top. Encourage children to sort their cubes based on which worker shows up on top after each roll. Repeat the rolling and sorting to help children identify all the workers.

MATERIALS

- one square cardboard box per child, photocopies of a wide range of health helper photographs or illustrations, and glue

OTHER IDEAS

- Show children puppets of health care workers, such as a doctor, a nurse, a dentist, a veterinarian, an optometrist, a paramedic, and so on. Invite children to use the puppets and tell everything they know about the health helper for which they have the puppet. Supplement information to ensure it is accurate and sufficient.

- Show children how to make a health helping-hands wreath by tracing their hand on photocopied photographs of health helpers, cutting out the outline of their hand on each page, and gluing the hands on a paper plate that has the center cut out.

- Read and discuss books on careers that include health helpers, such as *Career Day* by Anne Rockwell.

- Invite health professionals to visit the classroom and share what they do and where they work. Encourage each visitor to bring printed pictures, tools, and the clothes she uses for her job. Alternatively, video chat with a health professional, and ask for a virtual tour.

THE PEOPLE WHO HELP MY BODY STAY WELL! **37**

Accordion Book of Doctors and Nurses

Show children a variety of illustrations or photographs of doctors and nurses at work, and ask them what they think is happening in each image. Reinforce that doctors and nurses help you stay well through administering immunizations and help you heal when you are sick. Let them know that there are various kinds of doctors and that those who work mostly with children are called pediatricians. Assist children in creating an accordion-style book using multiple pieces of construction paper taped together to increase length and then folded back and forth. As an alternative to construction paper, use a strip of newspaper or chart paper. Allow children to select from doctor and nurse illustrations and photos provided, or locate additional ones. Help children measure so they can cut the images to fit their book pages and then glue them on each page. Provide a space where children can stand up their books for display.

MATERIALS

- magazine photos or illustrations downloaded from the Internet of doctors and nurses at work, construction paper, tape, and glue

OTHER IDEAS

- Read and discuss books about medical doctors and their jobs, such as *ABC Doctor: Staying Healthy from A to Z* by Liz Murphy, *Going to the Doctor* by Anne Civardi, and *Corduroy Goes to the Doctor* by Don Freeman.

- Teach children nursery rhymes and traditional songs, such as "Miss Polly Had a Dolly," "Five Little Monkeys Jumping on the Bed," "Jack and Jill," "Humpty Dumpty," and "It's Raining, It's Pouring," and discuss why characters in each one needed a doctor.

- Play, dance to, and listen to the words of songs related to going to the doctor, such as "Pop Fly," "Doctor, Doctor," "Sign My Cast," and "98.8" by Justin Roberts. Talk with children about when people need health helpers.

- Set up a doctor's office or medical clinic in the classroom, and add props to make it as realistic as possible. Help children make a sign for the office, set up a waiting room with toys or magazines, a reception desk, an exam table (a long coffee table), and a doctor's stool. Add a clipboard and pencil, a doctor's white coat or scrubs, empty medicine containers, a new unused syringe without the needle, a scale, a tape measure, a stethoscope, a reflex hammer, a blood pressure cuff, and other props. Include doctor-related photographs to inspire play.

Far and Near

When children are outside, ask them to face one direction and look at the things they can see, both close and far away. Write down the things they name. Provide tools to enhance sight (binoculars, magnifier, microscope, and telescope), and ask them to look again and describe what they see. Encourage them to give more detail about the same objects, as well as any new objects. Make a new list, and talk about the differences. Explain that we all use tools to help us see sometimes and that some people use these tools to see all the time. Show eyeglasses, and ask what the children know about them. Explain that eye doctors, who are called optometrists or ophthalmologists, use equipment to examine eyes and determine whether the person needs glasses and what strength of glasses.

MATERIALS

- paper, a marker, a magnifier, binoculars, a microscope, a telescope, a periscope, and a camera with a zoom lens

OTHER IDEAS

- To practice for an eye exam, give children a paper doll, and ask them to turn it like you are turning your paper doll. Hold the doll upright, to the left, upside down, and to the right. Try holding the paper doll at angles somewhere in between left, right, and upside down. Collect the paper dolls used by the children, and ask them to watch the way you turn your paper doll. Encourage them to use their fingers to point in the direction that the legs of the doll are pointing. These paper doll activities help children learn about direction.

- Provide an eye exam chart on a wall, a flashlight to highlight specific images on the chart, a paper cup to cover one eye when the other is being tested, a chair to sit in during the exam, and a yardstick to measure ten feet from the eye chart to the chair. Ask for a volunteer to sit in the chair and to point the direction of the E when it is highlighted with the flashlight. Let children know that an eye doctor sometimes uses other methods to check eyes, such as looking into them with a flashlight or asking people to wear special glasses and tell what they see.

■ Visit or invite an optometrist or ophthalmologist to the classroom, and ask him to explain his job, show tools or photographs of tools he uses, and demonstrate a quick eye exam. Request that he share with children how to take care of their eyes. Help children prepare questions in advance.

■ Set up an eye doctor's office in the classroom, and add props to make it as realistic as possible. Help children make a sign for the office and set up a waiting room with toys or magazines, a reception desk, an exam chair, and a doctor's stool. Add an adult's and a child's eye chart. Include a variety of eyeglass frames, some made by children and some contributed by an eye doctor's office.

A Hearing Test

Show children a bell, and ring it. Tell children to close their eyes and to raise both hands every time they hear the bell. Ring the bell loudly, moderately, and softly. When children open their eyes, tell them that some people have a hard time hearing sounds and may need special equipment or assistance. Since the people who have trouble hearing may not be aware of it, everyone should have hearing tests conducted by an audiologist. Read and discuss *Having a Hearing Test* by Vic Parker.

MATERIALS

■ a bell and *Having a Hearing Test* by Vic Parker

OTHER IDEAS

■ Visit or invite an audiologist to the classroom, and ask her to explain her job and show the tools (or photographs of tools) she uses. Request that she share with children how to take care of their ears. Help children come up with questions in advance.

■ Play and dance to "Let's Make Some Noise" by Raffi. Practice making low-, medium-, and high-pitched sounds, and explain that during a hearing exam some sounds may sound low, some medium, and others high.

■ Practice hearing exams by having children take turns using headphones. Ask children to raise their hands when they hear something. Turn music on, and slowly increase the volume as you watch for their signal.

■ Set up a hearing exam lab as a special interest area in the classroom, and add props to make it as realistic as possible. Help children make a sign for the office and set up a waiting room with toys or magazines, a reception desk, and an exam chair. Add headphones and items for creating sounds.

Visit the Dentist

Make arrangements for the children to visit a dental office. Independent dentists, dental clinics, mobile dental clinics, and dental hygiene schools are all potential learning sites. Before the visit, show children many photographs of things they may see, such as the patient chair, X-ray equipment and images, lights, dental instruments, and toothbrushes. During the visit, allow children to take photographs of the people working and the equipment they use. To ensure quality and variety, take some photos to add to those the children take. During the visit, make the experience as rich as possible. Children may find it interesting to see the dental instruments, an X-ray, tooth models, and the patient chair. Since children learn by being involved, encourage an active visit during which they can sit in the patient chair and touch a few selected objects, as well as learn about how the dentist can help them take care of their teeth. After the visit, assist the children in writing and illustrating an experience story to send as a thank-you. Use the photos taken to create a classroom book for children to look at and discuss their adventure.

MATERIALS

- cameras, large paper for the story, a marker, and art supplies for illustrations

OTHER IDEAS

- Add to the classroom a light table or light box and a variety of see-through objects, such as beads, frosted paper, acrylic tiles, sunglasses, tissue paper, plastic lids, and plastic drink bottles. Compare the light table to the X-ray machine the dentist used to look closely at teeth.

- Set up a dental clinic in the classroom, and add props to make it as realistic as possible. Help children make a sign for the office and set up a waiting room, a reception desk, a dental chair (reclining lawn chair), a doctor's white coat or scrubs, masks, gloves, and safety glasses for the dentist. Include dental-related photographs to inspire play.

- Give each child a two-liter soda bottle, and ask them to examine the bottom of it. (If two-liter soda bottles are not available, use water or juice bottles with a similar bottom.) Encourage each child to get the bottom of their bottle as dirty as they can. Provide soil, sand, and water, and encourage children to create mud to cover the bottom of their bottle. When children have their bottles dirty, label them and place them in a location to dry overnight. Once the bottles are dry, show children a clean one, and ask them to compare it to their molars. Explain that although they brush their teeth, it is hard to get them as clean as they need to be and that dental hygienists help people get their teeth really clean. Encourage them to be a dental hygienist and use a toothbrush to clean their "tooth" that they made dirty.

■ Puncture holes and cracks in the bottom of enough two-liter bottles for each child to have one. Show children the holes and cracks, and explain that sometimes teeth get cavities or break and need the help of a dentist. Encourage each child to fix their tooth, and provide playdough, glue, or a mixture of flour and water for them to use for their dental work.

Dogs Need Doctors Too

Read and discuss *Biscuit Visits the Doctor* by Alyssa Satin Capucilli or *Clifford Goes to the Doctor* by Norman Bridwell. Introduce the term *veterinarian*, and explain that these doctors are sometimes called *vets*. Invite any children who have gone with a pet to a vet visit to share their experience.

MATERIALS

- *Biscuit Visits the Doctor* by Alyssa Satin Capucilli or *Clifford Goes to the Doctor* by Norman Bridwell

OTHER IDEAS

- Hold up a series of toy animals from the classroom, one at a time, and ask what kind of animal it is and what kind of doctor it should go to if it is sick. Explain to children that veterinarians are doctors for many kinds of animals and that some vets treat pets, farm animals, zoo animals, racehorses, or even wild animals. Designate an area (box, rug, and so on), and engage children in looking throughout the room for other toy animals to bring to the designated spot. Help them name the animals, count the animals, and sort them into pet, farm, zoo, and other.

  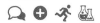

- Read and discuss books focused on what the job of the veterinarian is, such as *If I Were a Veterinarian* by Shelly Lyons and *A Day in the Life of a Veterinarian* by Heather Adamson.

- Visit, invite, or video chat with a veterinarian, and ask him to explain his job and show tools (or photographs of tools) he uses and any special clothes he wears. Request that he share with children how to take care of their pets. Help children prepare questions in advance.

  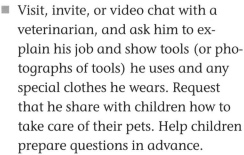

- Set up a veterinarian clinic in the classroom, and add props to make it as realistic as possible. Help children make a sign for the office and set up a waiting room, a reception desk, and an exam table. Include animal pictures and veterinarian-related pictures to inspire play. Add toy animals to the classroom to ensure there are plenty of patients.

FAMILY INFORMATION

THE PEOPLE WHO HELP MY BODY STAY WELL!

A visit to a doctor, dentist, or clinic is easier if your child knows what to expect. Talk to your child before going and help him or her understand that you are visiting a health helper. Take a favorite toy, a book, or crayons and paper along so your child can play while waiting for or receiving care. Holding a favorite doll or blanket often helps.

A child who is scared may not behave well. Talk about any fears your child may have. Try not to scare your child, but be honest. Assure your child that you will be there and will stay with her or him.

BE PREPARED

Before going to the doctor, make a list of your child's symptoms, such as fever, stomach pain, sore throat, coughing, or diarrhea. Behavior changes can also indicate health problems. Write down how long these symptoms have been present.

Learn what you can do to help your child. Ask questions such as the following:

- What is the name of the disease or condition? How long will it last?

- What medicine will my child need? Does the medicine have side effects?

- What other symptoms should I watch for, and how long will they last?

- Is the disease contagious? Can my child go back to school with this condition?

- Can this disease or condition be prevented?

FAMILY ACTIVITY

Help your child draw a line from each picture in the left column to the picture in the right column that shows the person who helps them care for that part of their body. Talk about who these people are and where they are located in your town, city, or community.

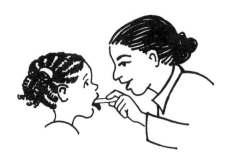

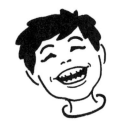

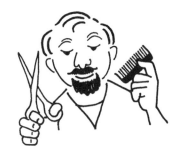

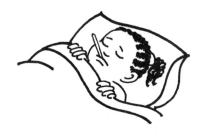

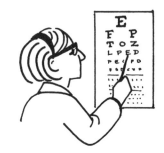

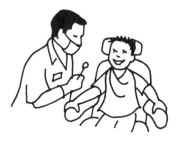

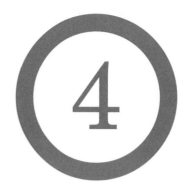

What I Have and Where It Comes From!

LEARNING OBJECTIVES

- Children will identify items that are needed every day (for example, food, clothes, shoes, soap, toothpaste).
- Children will begin to use the vocabulary of and recognize printed materials related to consumerism (for example, buy, sell, credit, shop, purchase, recycle, reuse).
- Children will identify ways to access health care and health care products.

Children use a wide range of items every day, both at home with their families and at school. From children's perspective, common items such as toilet paper and soap may simply "appear" in the bathroom. Many children haven't seen these items purchased in a store. Many children do, however, understand the concept of purchasing items such as candy or toys. You can talk with children to determine their frame of reference and build on their experiences.

When purchasing most items, consumers have a variety of choices. For example, a local store may have ten different brands of shampoo, and each of those brands may have five or more choices for fragrance, hair type, and color. Furthermore, there are various sizes of containers and prices for each. Likewise, food and beverage items include many choices. By making children aware that there are a variety of choices, you can help them identify products and services and the choices involved in making selections.

Food may be obtained from various sources. It can be purchased at grocery stores, farmers' markets, food co-ops, and restaurants or obtained through food banks and community gardens. Some families grow their own vegetables and herbs and have children help with that activity, and some children may have visited an orchard or farm and picked fresh produce (for example, apples, oranges, blueberries).

In addition to food, other products and necessities may be obtained from various sources. For example, clothing may be purchased or handmade, and gently used clothing is available through yard sales and consignment and thrift stores. Many community agencies and churches have clothing available for families in need. Children often enjoy getting hand-me-downs from older siblings, cousins, or friends. It can be a real treat for a child to receive a gently worn shirt from a special older friend!

Introduce services that are available, such as health care, and encourage children to talk about various health services and health care places they have visited. Children may have received vaccinations or other health services and dental services from doctors or other health care practitioners through private clinics, local health departments, hospitals, and mobile clinics, or through clinics set up in shopping centers and groceries and drugstores.

Newspaper and magazine advertisements, television commercials, and online websites can be used by teachers to introduce children to a wide range of available products and services. Discuss with children the many places to shop, such as malls, church-sponsored stores, flea markets, street vendors, consignment shops, Goodwill and Salvation Army stores, farmers' markets, yard sales, pawn shops, and online.

For older children, include in the discussions a variety of methods that might be used to obtain services or products. These include purchase orders, coins, paper money, gift certificates, credit, cash, checks, bartering, trading, food stamps, insurance cards, coupons, and debit cards. Many communities and even your classroom may include families who recently arrived from other countries. Some family members may travel internationally. As you study various methods of payment, encourage interest and discussion regarding currency from other countries.

Help children understand that many people make their own products, grow their own food, and use home health remedies (for example, lemon and honey for a cough). Others know how to repair broken items, such as repairing a flat tire or patching a hole in a favorite pair of pants. Encourage children to repair, reuse, and recycle items when appropriate.

VOCABULARY

advertisement	catalog	consignment	debit card
bar code	check	coupons	dime
cash	coins	credit card	discount

dollar	nickel	QR code	scanner
gift certificates	penny	quarter	
money order	price tag	receipt	
necessary	purchase	recycle	

CREATING THE ENVIRONMENT

- Allow children to set up a special store, clinic, or restaurant learning center so they can role-play being a consumer and making choices. As you gather clean empty packages and containers for classroom activities, be sure to include brands and items that children are likely to see in their own homes.

- Provide a variety of product and service advertisements, price tags, shopping lists, bills, receipts, ledgers, budgets, loan applications, play money, play credit cards, cash registers, phones, credit card machines, and boxes and shopping bags.

- Supply paper, poster board, and cardboard for children to use in making signs, billboards, and advertisements.

- Introduce currency from other countries, and use words from other languages to describe or name products and services.

EVALUATION

- Do children talk about the variety of items they use at home or at school?

- Are children role-playing and using a variety of words to describe obtaining and selling products and service?

- Do children role-play various ways to obtain products and services (including yard sales and trading)?

- In guided activities, can children recognize advertisements for products or services?

- During pretend play, do children demonstrate ways to obtain needed health care products or services?

CHILDREN'S ACTIVITIES

Shoes, Soap, and Soup

Show children bags and boxes holding food containers, clothing, and health-related products. Have each child select two items from the containers. Let children tell about their selections and why they picked those items. Help them identify necessary products used every day and products that may be desired but are not necessary. Encourage children to examine their selections to see any letters or words they recognize and to find a price tag to see the cost. Help them identify letters, words, and numbers.

❶ Safety Note: To avoid the danger of suffocation, supervise closely when plastic bags are used; remove them immediately at the conclusion of the activity.

MATERIALS
- bags (paper, plastic, and canvas), boxes, clothes (including shoes), food containers, containers for generic and name-brand health-related products (toothpaste, soap, shampoo, vitamins), and price tags on items

OTHER IDEAS

- Provide brand-name and generic containers of health care and hygiene products, and invite children to sort by type of product. Talk with children about the wide variety of brands and sizes from which people can choose when they are shopping. Ask how they would decide which toothpaste to buy. Explain that people may make choices based on size, price, taste, or fragrance or how well it works.

- Visit a store to see products children and their families use daily, and find out how much each costs. Look at price tags, and also place items under the customer scanner. Purchase an item, and let children observe the process.

- Show children several examples of QR codes and bar codes. Explain that these codes include information about what the product is and how much it costs. Engage children in creating bar codes and QR codes.

- Set up a store as a special interest area in the classroom, and add props to make it as realistic as possible. Provide a cash register, play money, calculators, and bags for purchases. Help children make a sign for the store, set up a checkout area, stock the shelves, make coupons, design advertisements, and hire staff. Engage children in creating products, like artwork or jewelry, to sell in the store on consignment.

Bag It, Box It

Exhibit a variety of shopping bags and boxes for children to describe and compare. Explain that when you buy something, you usually get a container in which to carry it, although some people bring their own containers as a way to reuse them. Let children open bags and unwrap empty health product containers that have been secured in newspaper or other protective wrap. Let children open boxes and find empty health product containers surrounded by various protective packing materials. Talk about what each packing material is, how it feels and smells, and why it might be used. Add protective packing materials to interest areas for further use as art supplies, to compare weights of materials, to determine if the materials float, to sort, and to haul in block area trucks.

❶ Safety Note: To avoid danger of suffocation or choking, supervise closely when using plastic bags, Styrofoam peanuts, Styrofoam blocks, foam, and Bubble Wrap. Remove plastic bags at the conclusion of the activity.

MATERIALS

- bags and boxes (large, medium, small, plastic, paper, canvas, netting, plain, colorful, with handles, without handles, for hang-up clothes, for shoes, for hats, for potatoes), protective packing materials (shredded and wadded newspaper, packing peanuts, foam blocks and inserts, corrugated cardboard, Bubble Wrap), and empty health product containers

OTHER IDEAS

- Go for a "bag walk" in a shopping center, and request a bag from several stores to display, study, and compare. Have the class vote on which is the most attractive, holds the most, is the strongest, and is most comfortable to carry.

- Invite a grocery store bagger to visit the classroom and demonstrate proper bagging of groceries. Ask the guest to explain the importance of placing items in the bags and how their jobs help consumers who are making purchases. Let children practice bagging as a follow-up.

- Provide children with paper bags and boxes, and encourage them to decorate creatively. Invite the children to produce a number of bags and boxes to be used in the classroom store.

■ Encourage children to make paper bag blocks by filling one paper bag with crumbled balls of newspaper and placing its open side down into another paper bag so both open ends are covered. Engage children in combining the paper bag blocks with boxes to create an obstacle course. Alter the course frequently.

Places to Shop

Prepare a slide show of many places to obtain products or services. Consider including photographs from a farmers' market, yard sale, pawn shop, consignment store, discount store, Goodwill store, Salvation Army store, street vendor, donation center, mall, public library, health department, military post exchange, and an ethnic grocery. Use photographs from local shopping options to help children identify with the shopping experience. After viewing the slide show, let children tell stories they have about shopping.

MATERIALS
- a camera, a viewing device, and a screen if needed

OTHER IDEAS

- Show children a variety of store advertisements and coupons. Explain what advertisements and coupons are. Encourage them to identify the store or product name for the advertisements and coupons you provide. Encourage children to identify letters, words, and numbers that are familiar to them, and provide information to support their early literacy efforts.

- Invite children's family members to visit and tell about places where they shop and why they choose to shop where they do, and to give examples of products they buy.

- Invite a business owner to visit the classroom and share information with the children about her products or service. Encourage the guest to bring examples of products or tools used for her service and to briefly discuss pricing.

- Read and discuss books about family-owned businesses, such as *Grandpa's Corner Store* by DyAnne DiSalvo-Ryan.

Mail Order and More

Let children know that not everyone goes to a store to purchase what they need or want. Show children a wide range of printed catalogs, including those for clothing, health products, food, toys, tools, seeds and plants, and preschool classroom supplies. Encourage children to look through the catalogs and identify categories of things they use every day, locate the item numbers, and check prices. Show them the order forms, and explain that one way to shop is to fill out the form with the item number and description and mail the order form or call the company to place an order. Provide copies of the order forms for children to use in role-playing how to order materials from a catalog.

MATERIALS
- a wide range of catalogs, copies of order forms, and toy or old telephones (remove the batteries from cell phones)

OTHER IDEAS
- Provide a catalog order form for a small group, and encourage every child to use a black fine-tip marker to write or draw something on the form. Tell children that some people fax the order form to buy products instead of mailing it. Show children a fax machine, and send the page to a predetermined location. Arrange for someone to send a fax back with a message to the children so they can watch the receipt.

- Explain to children that some people shop by ordering from television shows. Show children a short segment of a shopping show, and explain that when people watching find something they like, they can make a telephone call and order it.

Let children know that people sometimes make a telephone call to order products from catalogs. Demonstrate for the children how to order an item, and provide toy or unconnected telephones for children to role-play ordering.

- Show children an online shopping site that includes children's toys and books. Explain that it is a catalog on the Internet. Allow children to help choose a product to order for the classroom. Demonstrate how to proceed through the ordering process, even if you are not placing an order at that time. Let children see the icon for the shopping cart to familiarize them with the process.

■ Tell children that in addition to shopping in stores or catalogs, some people shop when they attend shopping parties in the homes of others. Invite someone who sells products through home parties to throw a miniparty for the classroom and explain to the children his job, his products, and pricing. Examples include representatives of Avon, Pampered Chef, Usborne Books, Mary Kay, and Discovery Toys.

Ways to Pay

Display coin banks, and give each child some coins to put in them. Let children tell you what they know about money. Ask what people do with money. See if they know about ways to purchase items other than by using money. Show a container with various methods of payment represented (see materials list). Tell the children that sometimes people use cash to pay for products and services, and sometimes they use other ways to pay. Let children examine the items and talk about them. Explain that you are going to use them for a bulletin board exhibit and want them to help you create the exhibit.

MATERIALS

- coin banks, coins, a container, simulated or expired methods of payment (gift certificates, gift cards, coupons, tokens, barter agreements, credit cards, debit cards, checks, coins, dollar bills, foreign currency, insurance cards, medical cards, library cards, gas cards, and so on), and adhesive for securing payment methods to a bulletin board

OTHER IDEAS

- Visit a bank and explore the machines and what people who work there do.

- Invite guests to show and tell about money from other countries.

- Read and discuss books that include money language, such as *The Big*

Green Pocketbook by Candice Ransom and *One Cent, Two Cents, Old Cent, New Cent: All About Money* by Bonnie Worth.

- Play songs with money language, such as "Magic Penny" by Tickle Tune Typhoon.

Grow, Create, Repair, and Reuse

Show children produce from a garden, homemade materials, items in need of repair, and secondhand items. Explain that sometimes things can be grown in your own garden, be homemade, be fixed, or be used secondhand instead of purchased new. Invite discussion about children's experiences with gardening, creating, cleaning, repairing, loaning, and receiving secondhand items. Accept and show respect for all children's stories, and guide the discussion in nonjudgmental ways.

MATERIALS

- garden produce, shoes in need of repair, garments missing a button or with a small hole, a clothing pattern, handmade toys, and secondhand clothes and other items

OTHER IDEAS

- Play and move to "Down on Grandpa's Farm" by Raffi. Talk about how growing your own food saves money and gives you healthier food too.

- Visit a shoe, clock, or auto repair shop, or have a repair person visit the classroom and demonstrate how to use tools of the trade. Alternatively, watch a short video clip of a person making a repair. Help children learn about the skills for fixing things and the value of fixing something instead of replacing it.

- Visit a seamstress, tailor, or alteration shop, or have a representative visit the classroom and demonstrate a little about her job. Or invite a shop to video chat with the class.

- Set up a consignment store as a special interest area in the classroom, and add props to make it as realistic as possible. Engage children in making products to sell in the store.

FAMILY INFORMATION

WHAT I HAVE AND WHERE IT COMES FROM!

Children use a wide variety of items every day, both at home and at school. Include your child when you shop as a way to model decision making. As you select items to purchase, talk about what you are buying and why. This will help children see that adults make choices about what they buy, rather than buying everything on the shelf.

Ask your child to help you select health-related products, such as soap, shampoo, or toothpaste. You can discuss how you use them; select the scent, flavor, or color you prefer; and compare the prices of various brands. Promote a feeling of independence by allowing your child to choose a product from the shelf, such as colorful bandages or his or her favorite toothpaste.

WHERE FOOD COMES FROM

Children may be more likely to try a new food if they help select it. Some children have fruits and vegetables growing in their own yard, but there are many children who do not know that apples grow on trees and potatoes grow in the ground.

Take your child to visit various places where food is available. Some examples are the produce aisle of a grocery store, farmers' markets, and pick-your-own orchards and berry fields. Look at the various colors, shapes, and sizes of produce, and let your child help select your purchase.

If possible, grow your own foods. Lettuce, radishes, strawberries, and herbs can grow quickly in pots. If you have a sunny area for a garden, try tomatoes, potatoes, eggplant, or other fruits and vegetables.

FAMILY ACTIVITY

Attach the sheet below to cardboard, and then cut out the puzzle pieces. While working the puzzle, talk with your child about how we get the food, clothing, personal care products, and so on that we need. Who or what makes them and where? Where do they go after they are made? How do they get to your home? You may wish to discuss the difference between shops and farmers' markets, and how some people make their own clothes, grow their own food, and so on.

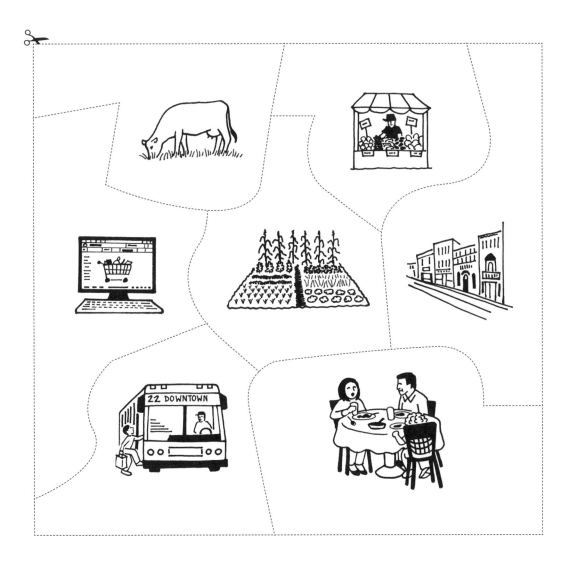

Helping My Family and Friends!

LEARNING OBJECTIVES

- Children will communicate ways each family member helps at home.

- Children will identify ways they can help at home.

- Children will practice helping behaviors in the classroom.

Every family is special. Families may be different in structure (for example, one or two parents, blended families, foster families), and individual roles and responsibilities may vary. Families also have similarities. For example, every family will have someone who helps prepare meals, whether it is the mother, father, grandmother, older sibling, or outside help.

Children are familiar with the roles each of their own family members play, and they may become confused as they discover that roles vary in other families. Encourage children to share with the class how their family members help one another at home. This allows children to discover similarities and differences in roles and to identify the variety of ways people help one another.

Encourage children to explore and discuss ways they can help at home. Developing self-help skills as they learn to take care of their dressing needs in order to use the bathroom and to prepare for outside play is one way they help at home. Children may have specific responsibilities, such as feeding pets, emptying trash baskets, and putting away toys. With adult supervision, children may help with younger siblings in the family. Young children can place napkins or eating utensils on the table for meals; older children may assist with serving food or pouring beverages.

Although there are individual differences, many children like to do things for themselves because it makes them feel good. Children may enjoy helping others if it is proposed in a positive way and the task is not too overwhelming. Some children may find it difficult to accept help from others and may see the help provided to them as taking away their freedom or power. Understanding each child's personality is important as you encourage development of cooperation and social skills.

Also, be familiar with cultural and personal preferences within families. Some cultures do not encourage self-help responsibilities for young children, such as dressing oneself or learning to self-serve foods. At school, children may need to develop independence skills due to the staff ratio and curriculum goals; however, respect should be shown for families whose practices emphasize caretaking and responsibility to the group over self.

In the classroom, acknowledge children's efforts to dispose of trash, put away toys, and dress themselves for outdoor play. Encourage development of cooperation skills as children work together in pretend play and prepare for mealtime (for example, getting napkins and eating utensils). During outside play, help children learn to take turns (for example, only one child climbing the slide ladder at a time), and help children learn to play together by suggesting activities that can be enjoyed by two or more children.

Children can help one another feel better by using kind words, playing together, and sharing ideas and interests. Chores in the classroom can be shared to reinforce helping.

VOCABULARY

appreciation	dust	Laundromat	shared
attic	greeting cards	outside	shoveling
basement	handy	pay	tools
chores	helping hand	rescue	utility
cleanup	hire	responsibilities	
contribute	inside	rotate	
cooperate	jobs	scratch	

CREATING THE ENVIRONMENT

■ Provide books that show nonsexist roles for family members and a variety of helping behaviors to help children see and accept differences.

■ Design an environment that encourages children to act independently when selecting toys and returning them. Easily accessible, low shelves promote children's returning materials and toys to their appropriate place.

- Supply props for role-playing cleaning in dramatic play, and materials for making things for people in the woodworking and art areas.

- Encourage children to prepare thank-you notes when people help them by providing paper and a variety of writing tools in the language arts center.

- Incorporate pets and plants into the classroom, and allow children to assist with their care to give children an opportunity to practice helping behaviors.

EVALUATION

- Do children talk about jobs their family members do to be helpful at home (take out trash, cook meals, water plants, and feed pets)?

- During pretend play focused on home and family, do children role-play a variety of helpful behaviors?

- Do children help with meal service (for example, set table, throw away trash)?

- Do children increasingly initiate helping activities at school (for example, put away toys)?

- Do children discuss ways people help each other (for example, help lift a heavy object, give a drink of water, help tie shoes)?

CHILDREN'S ACTIVITIES

Who in the Family Does It?

In a group, ask children to generate a list of jobs people do at home as you write each one on chart paper. Ask children to tell who in their home does each job. Add the person mentioned beside the items or jobs on the list, or create a chart listing titles of people across the top (daddy, mom, dad's partner, mom's partner, stepmother, stepfather, uncle, aunt, auntie, grandmother, grandfather, big sister, little brother, cousin, or any other person represented in children's families) and the jobs down the left side. Put a check in the job's row under the person's title when a child mentions that this person does a particular job at her or his house. Remind children that both men and women can do the various chores, and point out that in some situations chores are shared or rotated, or someone outside the family is hired to do it. Help children see as much variety as possible in roles and responsibilities.

MATERIALS
- chart paper and markers

OTHER IDEAS

- Play, sing, and discuss songs about family roles, such as "Shoveling" by the Cat's Pajamas, "Stay-at-Home Dad," "My Brother Did It," and "From Scratch" by Justin Roberts.

- Invite family members of enrolled children, friends, and coworkers to talk about roles and show photographs of them doing chores in their family. Include a variety of families so that children can see and appreciate diversity in people and helping roles.

- Read and discuss a variety of books showing family roles, such as *Daddy Makes the Best Spaghetti* by Anna Grossnickle Hines and *Mommy, Mama, and Me* by Lesléa Newman.

- Explain that families may pay someone outside of the family to do some jobs, or trade jobs with someone in another family. Invite a professional house cleaner or "fix-it" person to come into the classroom and tell about how he takes care of what families need done. Encourage the guest to show some of the tools he uses when doing his job or show before and after photographs.

Helping on the Inside

Show children a dollhouse, complete with furniture, or a detailed photograph of the inside of a dollhouse. Point to one room at a time, and ask children what that room is named. Let them know if other titles are sometimes given to such a room (den, family room, playroom, living room, and so on). Encourage children to identify the furniture and other things in each room and to share what they think children may play in each room. See if children know of other rooms some houses have that the dollhouse does not, such as an office, sunroom, laundry or utility room, basement, garage, attic, or hall. Tell children that all rooms in a home need to be taken care of and cleaned. Ask children to act out ways they could be helpful in each room, and let others guess what the helpful act is. Write down the helpful ideas children offer, and make suggestions to supplement theirs. Children whose living space is not similar to the dollhouse may become anxious and need reassurance that it is okay if their living space is different from the dollhouse or other children's homes. Help them see that everyone can be helpful in her living space.

MATERIALS

- dollhouse or a photograph of the inside of a dollhouse, chart paper, and markers

OTHER IDEAS

- Help children develop a chart to take home for keeping track of ways they help inside.

- Invite older siblings of the enrolled children to visit the classroom and describe a chore they do at home, show photographs or a video of doing the chore, and explain why it is important.

- Tell children that sometimes people help in homes that are not their own, and ask if they have any examples to share. Read and discuss *The Berenstain Bears Lend a Helping Hand* by Stan and Jan Berenstain.

- Ask children if they have ever been helpful in a store. Read and talk about *Feast for 10* by Cathryn Falwell.

Helping Outside

Ask children to think about and give examples of spaces they might find outside where they live (apartment court, front steps, front gate, backyard, garage, storage building, porch, patio, deck, swimming pool, garden, gazebo, rooftop, alley, driveway). Help children understand that some people have yards and others do not. Listen carefully, and make a list as children give examples of spaces found outside their home. Encourage children to describe how they play in any of those areas. Ask children what kinds of chores have to be done for each of these spaces. Write beside each space the chores children mention. Review the lists with the children, and ask them which of the chores they could help someone do.

MATERIALS
- chart paper and markers

OTHER IDEAS

- Help the children develop a chart to take home and use in tracking things they can help with outside.

- Read *My Steps* by Sally Derby. Ask children if they have ideas about how to keep the steps clean so that children can continue to play there.

- Ask children if they know of ways to be helpful other than cleanup chores. Read books that give helpful examples beyond cleaning, such as *Hana Rescues Misty* by Azra Z. Mehdi and *Herman the Helper* by Robert Kraus.

- Teach children songs about being helpful, such as "If I Had a Hammer," written by Pete Seeger and Lee Hays, or songs about working, such as "I've Been Working on the Railroad."

How Does It Work?

Gather several items used for cleaning or maintaining home living space. Assist small groups of children in disassembling and assembling various parts of these items. Show children how to install new bags and filters on vacuums or empty canisters, how to change sponges or wipes on mops, how to add cord to the weed trimmer, how to empty the hand vacuum, how to change batteries in flashlights, and how to change the faucet aerator.

MATERIALS

■ vacuum cleaners, vacuum bags and filters, weed trimmers and cord, sponge mops and sponges, rags, flashlights and batteries, a faucet and aerator, and hand tools necessary for disassembling these items (screwdrivers, wrenches)

OTHER IDEAS

■ Engage children in sorting doll clothes and dress-up clothes by color. Talk about the importance of clean clothes. Visit a laundry room or laundromat, and demonstrate the various knobs and parts of the washing machines and dryers. Show children where the water hoses and lint traps are, and explain how to clean components to increase the life of the machines.

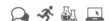

■ Provide old clocks, lamps, and other materials children can disassemble while learning to use tools.

■ Play "Humpty Dumpty" by the Cat's Pajamas, and explain that not everything can always be fixed but that many things can be. Visit a repair shop, and observe the activity, or invite a repair person to visit the classroom. Ask the repair person to explain her job and show items that she has fixed.

■ Read and discuss *Mighty Mike Repairs a Playground* by Kelly Lynch.

Handy Helper

Explain to children that they are each going to make a "Handy Helper" box and fill it with "Handy Helper" items. Have each child choose a box and use art supplies to add interesting and personal touches. Assist children in attaching string handles, cutting handholds, or designing a lid for their box or container. Add the children's names to their boxes, or let them write their names on their boxes. Provide a selection of nontoxic cleaning supplies for children to select from to supply their boxes.

MATERIALS

- shoe box–size boxes, art supplies, and a variety of nontoxic cleaning supplies (clean rags, old socks, sponges, yarn, string, spray bottles [clean and empty], cloths, paper bags, plastic scrubbers, gloves)

OTHER IDEAS

- Show children a variety of tools, including dust rags, and read *Tools* by Ann Morris.

- Visit a hardware store or a variety store to see the various types of cleaning supplies and tools they have for helping inside, outside, and all about.

- Read *You Make Me Happy* by Laurie Barrows. Explain that some chores are better done together, but sometimes adults need to do chores and the children's job is to play independently.

- Remind children that helping includes many activities, like bringing someone water when he is sick, sending a card to someone who is sad, or giving a gift to someone who is lonely. Show children some examples of greeting cards, and encourage children to create some greeting cards to go into their Handy Helper box.

Helping at School

Develop a reusable chart for daily classroom and playground chores. Each day, invite children to form friendship teams or pairs, assisting as needed so that everyone is included. Ask each team or pair to choose a classroom chore to work on together. After completing their daily chore, they can add a mark, star, or other designation to the chart. Talk with children about how they play together, but sometimes they work together too.

MATERIALS
- reusable chart and a marker

OTHER IDEAS

- Explain to children that when someone helps them, it is polite to say thank you and show appreciation. Let them know that people can say thank you with words out loud or with written words, as in a card. Encourage children to practice saying thank you and to create some thank-you cards that they can give to each other and to family members when someone helps them.

- Invite a variety of program employees to visit the classroom and describe for children how they help the children, parents, teachers, and others at the school. Encourage the guests to give examples, provide pho-tographs, and show any tools they use to help others.

- Read and talk about *Horton Hears a Who!* by Dr. Seuss, and talk about the importance of being helpful and standing up for (advocating for) others.

- Play "Help!" by the Beatles. Tell children that they should try to do things that need to be taken care of, but when they need help, they should ask for it. And when they see that someone else needs help, they should see if they can be helpful.

FAMILY INFORMATION

HELPING MY FAMILY AND FRIENDS!

Children like to do things they see their family members do. Your child can watch and learn to help with simple chores, such as folding clothes or setting the table. These can be fun activities that help your child develop skills. Gather writing materials, and sit down with your child. Together you can create a list of things your child can do to help around the house. Encourage your child to assist with putting away pots and pans, taking care of pets, matching socks, planting or weeding flowers, washing the car, dusting, mopping, raking leaves, painting a fence or a room, cleaning up the yard, watering plants, or assembling shelves or furniture.

Your child can help at home and develop self-help skills while learning to take care of his or her dressing needs in order to use the bathroom and to prepare for outside play. These activities help your child develop independence and decision-making skills too.

LEARNING NEW SKILLS

Each time your child tries to help, acknowledge her or his efforts by saying something like, "I like it when you help" or "Thank you for helping." This builds confidence and helps your child want to keep helping.

Please have lots of patience as your child learns to help. Children's work will not be complete or perfect. Your child may lose interest in an activity after just a few minutes. Try to break chores into smaller or shorter activities that allow for success and frequent stops and starts.

FAMILY ACTIVITY

With your child, look at each of the pictures below, and discuss what children are doing to help in each one. Talk about additional ways children can and do help their friends and family and, specifically, ways your child helps out.

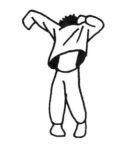 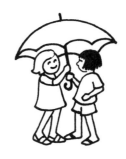

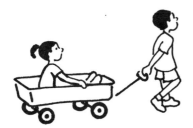 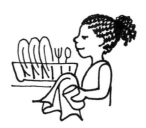

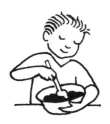 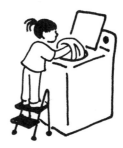

 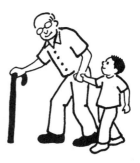

Taking Care of My Places and Spaces!

LEARNING OBJECTIVES

- Children will identify various environments (for example, classroom, playground, street, and home).

- Children will identify specific places in their environment (for example, a bedroom or kitchen within their house, their classroom within the school).

- Children will pick up trash, put away toys and tools, and care for plants and animals.

An environment is a surrounding area, such as one's home, the school and classroom, a playground or park, and the street on which one lives. Since people are very mobile, children experience being in many environments each day. Do not expect children to completely understand or be able to define the term *environment*. With appropriate use and learning activities, however, children should be able to recognize various environments or areas with which they are familiar.

Young children cannot comprehend an environment beyond that which they can see. A child who has never seen a pond, lake, river, or ocean cannot comprehend a large area of water with fish and other living creatures. Therefore, it is not appropriate to talk about water pollution as a global idea and expect children to comprehend what that means. They can, however, understand that a fishbowl or aquarium is an environment with living creatures. If there is a body of water in your area, children can understand keeping that specific environment clean since they can see it.

Whereas older children can recognize that their home and street are part of a larger community, younger children can relate only to their own home and other homes they see around them. As children recognize which bedroom, house, classroom, or playground is theirs, work with them to learn how to take care of their toys, pets, or other items in the home environment. Talk with them about how they (and you!) are taking care of the classroom environment when we put toys away after using them and put trash in the garbage can. As children grow older, talk about ways to care for their larger environments (neighborhoods), such as by recycling, planting flowers and trees, and putting trash where it belongs.

Children begin helping their environment as they become familiar with the expectations for their school and classroom experience. Thank children for efforts in disposing of trash and putting away toys and puzzles. On the playground, invite one or two children to help you each day by pointing out trash; only adults should pick up trash and debris on the playground.

Help children learn to reduce waste by reusing and recycling. Reuse paper by drawing on both sides of the page; use broken crayons, which still work for coloring; and recycle vegetable and fruit peelings by composting. Shredded newspaper may provide bedding for pet cages, while crumpled paper provides cushioning for packing breakable items. Model conservation by turning the tap water off while brushing your teeth. Encourage children to share their ideas for reducing waste, reusing, and recycling.

VOCABULARY

air	extinct	pollution	waste
climate	forest	recycle	water
conservation	globe	renewable	wilderness
earth	green	reuse	world
ecology	land	sanitation	
energy	litter	solar	
environment	nature	sustainability	

CREATING THE ENVIRONMENT

- Include opportunities to practice caring for the various environments with which children come into contact. Model conservation, recycling, reusing, and beautification to help children attach concrete actions to the concepts of caring for the environment. Teacher modeling may include showing children how to use water wisely, reusing or recycling materials from home for various learning centers, collecting other materials to take to recycling centers, and adding plants and pictures to the classroom.

- Provide a fish tank in the classroom so that children who do not live close to a body of water can learn about keeping water clean.

■ Acquire a classroom pet so that children can assist with the care and cleaning of its space and witness how environments affect living things.

EVALUATION

■ Do children talk about their environment?

■ Can children identify various environments (for example, classroom, playground, home, park)?

■ Can children identify specific areas of their environment (for example, classroom, restroom, or cafeteria within their school)?

■ Does role playing relate to taking care of the environment?

■ Do children increasingly initiate actions to help the environment (for example, pick up toys, recycle)?

CHILDREN'S ACTIVITIES

In My World

Ask children to draw pictures or make clay representations of something in a place that is special to them. Let children know that a special place may be a bedroom, a hallway, a play space, the backseat of a car, a toy box, or wherever they keep some of their things. After displaying their completed work to the group, ask them to tell about it. As each thing is named, ask how they take care of that item ("How do you take care of your bed?" "How do you take care of your clothes?" "How do you take care of your stuffed animal?").

MATERIALS

- paper, art supplies, and clay

OTHER IDEAS

- Ask children to draw pictures of things outside their home or living space. Ask the same kinds of questions ("How do you take care of . . . ?") regarding such things as trees, cars, plants, animals, buildings, sidewalks, and grass.

- Have each child trace an object from school and then make a mosaic by gluing small pieces of cut paper inside the outline of the object. Discuss with children how to care for the object they traced.

- Invite children to pick an object in the classroom or at home and make up a poem or story about where it came from. After each child shares his or her poem or story, discuss the care of the object.

- Read and discuss books such as *All Around Me I See* by Laya Steinberg, *Home* by Jeannie Baker, and *Our Big Home: An Earth Poem* by Linda Glaser.

  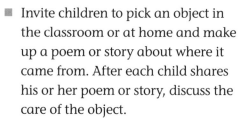

Respect My Space

Have children pick an item from the classroom that they are going to be responsible for, care for, clean, or organize. Ask children to think about how they will be responsible for the item, and then record them explaining their plan for cleaning, organizing, or caring for what they have chosen. After they have carried out their plan, have children report about their experience and share whether they followed their recorded plans.

 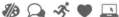

MATERIALS
- audio recording device and a player

OTHER IDEAS
- Read and discuss *Home* by Jeannie Baker.

- Take the class to volunteer at a food bank or co-op, at Goodwill or Salvation Army, or at a plant nursery or botanical gardens. Before the trip, talk about how each of these places helps take care of people and the earth's resources by working cooperatively, recycling, renewing, or reusing. While there, children might help put away supplies, water plants, fold and help put clothes in storage, or organize items for display.

- Read and discuss *City Green* by Dy-Anne DiSalvo-Ryan.

- Play and move to "Turn the World Around" by Music for the Little People Kids Choir.

Don't Waste It, Dump It, or Pollute It

Visit a recycling center or a waste collection site or facility. Prepare the children for the visit by reading stories or reference materials that describe such places. Look at photographs or short video clips of these kinds of places, and encourage children to share what they know about them. During the field trip, ask children to identify items they see that have been sent to be recycled at the recycling center or that have been dumped at the landfill.

MATERIALS

- stories and reference materials that include information about landfills, recycling centers, and pollution

OTHER IDEAS

- Read and discuss *Smash! Mash! Crash! There Goes the Trash!* by Barbara Odanaka.

- Read and discuss *Where Once There Was a Wood* by Denise Fleming.

- Invite people who work at a recycling center or waste collection site or facility to visit or video chat and talk about their jobs.

- Watch, sing along to, and dance to the "Reduce, Reuse, Recycle," video on YouTube at http://www.youtube .com/watch?v=sQoM9aAtfvc, or search the Internet for songs about reduce, reuse, and recycle to share with the children.

Stash the Trash

After talking about recycling with the children, ask them to suggest items that can be recycled or reused. Make a list of their suggestions, and ask which items might be found in the classroom. Choose a trash container that is least likely to present health risks, and conduct an examination of current classroom trash. Demonstrate proper trash handling by wearing gloves, glasses, and an apron and by washing your hands after handling the trash. Let children put on gloves and goggles or protective glasses and examine the trash from the selected container. As each item is handled, ask whether it could be recycled or reused. Add the items that children suggest to the list of recyclables and reusables.

Ask the children for ideas about how to sort and classify materials to be recycled. Allow children to create a recycling plan, and help them think of supplies needed to carry it out. Let the children put their plan into action. Help them find the needed supplies to prevent spilling and to label bags, boxes, and containers. Help children determine where to take items for recycling. Remind children to wash their hands after handling the used items and to wear protective gloves when they sort trash.

MATERIALS
■ boxes and bags, bag ties, tape, markers, blank paper, newsprint, gloves, goggles, aprons, other protective clothing, a wagon or rolling cart, and water for cleaning up

OTHER IDEAS
■ After examining items from the trash (taking precautions as mentioned above), help children decide which items might be reused in interest areas or elsewhere in the classroom, how the items will be reused, and how they can be cleaned or sanitized before reuse.

■ Read and discuss *The Three R's: Reuse, Reduce, Recycle* by Nuria Roca.

■ Play, sing along with, and dance to "Conviction of the Heart" by Kenny Loggins.

■ After learning about recycling, plan a "cleanup day" with the children for either the classroom, an area of the playground, or a nearby park. Ask the children what items they think will be needed for "cleanup day," and help them create a list. Be sure to have gloves and other protective gear, bins for sorting, and time to "wash up" after "cleanup." Remember that adults should pick up the trash.

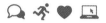

Teaching Others

After children have visited a recycling center or learned about recycling, have them discuss things they would say to help other people learn how to recycle. During the discussion, take careful notes regarding their ideas. Ask them to role-play their ideas. After they have practiced and role-played, create a video of the children teaching about recycling. Have the children watch the video, and reshoot or make another if they would like to improve on their technique. The final version can be introduced to other classes, shown at an open house or at community events, or sent to a local television station. Remember to obtain parent permission prior to their child's image or name being included for media purposes, including social media such as Facebook.

MATERIALS

■ a video camera, a video-watching device, props and costumes, markers, chart paper, and photographs or signs about recycling

OTHER IDEAS

■ Divide children into groups, and have them role-play teaching various environmental concepts they have learned about, such as "don't pollute," "don't waste," "clean up your mess," "recycle and reuse," "dumping is dirty," and "take care of your space." Allow children to help with making the video.

■ Play, sing along to, and dance to "Garbage Blues" by Tickle Tune Typhoon.

■ Play, sing, and discuss the song "Shoveling" by Tom Chapin.

■ Provide materials (markers, poster board, old magazines, and so on), and encourage children, either individually or in groups, to make "Healthy Environment" posters that help people learn to dispose of their trash properly, recycle, clean up inside and outside spaces, reduce use of water and energy, and so on.

Reduce and Renew

Read to children the suggested titles in the materials list or in other books about taking care of the earth, and talk about the various ways mentioned to nurture the environment. Help children discover ways to "care for the earth," such as reducing the water we use by turning off the faucet while we brush or "lather up," planting trees and improving green spaces to help purify the air we breathe and to provide shade and insulation to reduce the energy we use, and choosing to use renewable energies such as wind and solar power.

MATERIALS

- *The Earth and I* by Frank Asch, *Michael Recycle* by Ellie Bethel, or *I Can Save the Earth! One Little Monster Learns to Reduce, Reuse and Recycle* by Alison Inches, and access to a library or the Internet for research

OTHER IDEAS

- Encourage children to dress up and role play one of the stories in a book you have read about caring for the earth. Video or photograph the activity, and play it at a parents'/family meeting or event, or make individual photographs available to families.

- Help children write letters or e-mail messages to environmental groups to request information.

- Assist children in making a list of rhyming words related to reducing waste and recycling, and help them use these rhyming words to craft a song they can sing to familiar tunes such as "Itsy Bitsy Spider" and "Twinkle, Twinkle Little Star."

- Help children research how plants contribute to the air we breathe, and dedicate a time for "planting something green" in the classroom or on the playground/school grounds.

FAMILY INFORMATION

TAKING CARE OF MY PLACES AND SPACES!

As children begin to recognize which bedroom, house, or yard is theirs, work with them to learn to take care of their toys, pets, or other items in the home environment. Talk with your child about how we are taking care of our environment when we put away our toys after we use them and when we put our trash in the garbage can.

With help from your child, plant a tree in your backyard, add live flowers to a room or garden, or clean some part of your home. Talk about how this makes your environment more appealing and a nice place to be.

Children can learn to recycle and reuse through everyday home activities. Broken toys can be mended, paper can be colored on both sides, and clothes can be handed down when children have outgrown them.

Find out what reuse and recycling services are available in your community. Set up recycling containers, bins, boxes, or bags, with help and information supplied by your child.

OUR COMMUNITY ENVIRONMENT

As children grow older, they will learn that their home and school environments are part of a larger environment, such as a neighborhood or community. Talk about ways to care for these environments, such as by recycling, planting flowers and trees, and putting trash where it belongs.

FAMILY ACTIVITY

Encourage your child to color the picture below as you discuss the benefits of recycling and how trash hurts our environment. Together, create a plan for how your child can help with recycling and cleaning up or improving the environment.

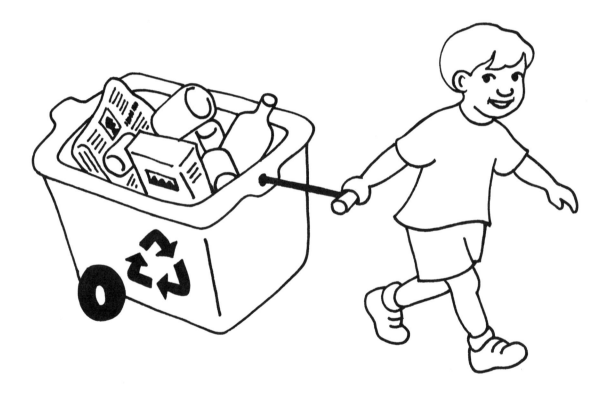